John Hope Navigates

THE DIAMOND PENDANT

Adventures for Seniors

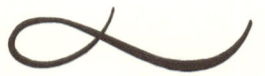

seniorality

John Hope Navigates The Diamond Pendant - John Hope, Michael L. Mann

Copyright © 2024 Seniorality / Everbreeze Media Oy

This is a work of fiction. Names and characters are the product of the author's imagination and any resemblance to actual persons, living or dead, is entirely coincidental.

Set in 22 pt EB Garamond

Chapter 1
Boat Repairs

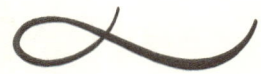

I'VE ALWAYS thought that yachts seem lonely when they are out of the water, and 'Morning Mist' was no exception.

Stepping down next to the boat cradle, I gazed up at her hull, now freshly washed and clean of seaweed and other marine dirt. Smooth and rounded, the hull invited my touch. I absent-mindedly ran my hand along its curve, like a father guiding a nervous child on its first day of school.

The yacht had been hoisted out of the water onto the boat cradle three days earlier. Despite my extensive shipyard experience, I couldn't shake off my anxiety whenever a boat was on land.

Since then, I had meticulously supervised the yacht's repairs, scrutinizing each fix and repair to ensure they met my exacting standards.

Late in the afternoon, as I emerged from the bilge into the engine room, I banged my head on the beam. "Ouch!" I moaned, rubbing my head with a grubby hand.

"Watch yourself, John. Gotta take better care of what's left in there," Captain Remington quipped, opening the engine room door.

"Hell, Remy, you nearly gave me a heart attack. Wasn't expecting you 'til five, but it's damn good to see you. You're looking fit and tanned," I exclaimed.

"I've been on break for the past couple of weeks, John. Your call came at the perfect time. I start feeling jittery if I spend too long on land. Need the sea air to keep me sane. And you John, you're looking sharp, aside from that bump on your noggin," Remy asked with a grin.

"Let's grab a beer and sit down. I've had my fill for the day. You head on over to the aft deck, I'll hit a quick shower and then catch up with you," I said.

Captain Remington grabbed a couple of beers from the refrigerator and strolled through the saloon to the rear aft deck.

The saloon exuded an air of casual elegance — cream-colored, plush couches encircling a polished mahogany coffee table, with a small library nestled against the aft bulkhead. Double doors beckoned toward the aft deck, where a collection of cane chairs surrounded a teak table. How many leisurely lunches had we shared in this very spot? He smiled to himself as the memories flooded back.

Seated there, he pondered if there could ever be a more picturesque view: crystal-clear Bahamas water sparkling under the late afternoon sun and rippled by the faintest of breezes.

Captain Remington smiled as he reminisced about the many years we had sailed alongside each other. How long had we known each other? Since those early days of diving together to inspect yacht blocks during docking. We had been armed with nothing but goggles and fins—no air tanks needed. I could hold my breath longer than anyone Remington knew.

I joined Remy in the saloon and together we recalled the first time I had assisted Remy in lifting a yacht out of the water.

"Remember Remy" I had said, "a yacht is like an egg standing upright in the water. Remove the water, and the egg topples over. Yachts behave the same; it's our duty to ensure they remain steady," I had explained to him. It was a rule that had stuck with Remington through the years.

It was my nature to always be direct and I was known to be a straight talker. If something needed to be done, I usually found the energy to make it happen.

Against the odds, I had built an enviable reputation as a shipyard expert and those that knew me, respected my abilities in a tight spot, be it on land or at sea.

Yet I think Remington now noticed a softer and more mellow side to me. The years of experience had definitely tempered me, instilling a more thoughtful approach to challenges, a departure from my earlier, gun-ho attitude.

"Cheers, Remy. Gorgeous water today, huh?" I said, taking a seat across the table from my old friend, my short blonde hair still damp from the shower.

"Sitting here, gazing out at Paradise Island, I never tire of this view. Even better when it's not peak holiday season."

I took a sip from my beer and then continued, "Sylvia let me know she and the interior decorator will arrive on Friday. I told her she'll have to coordinate with you; I'm not the best at dealing with the decorating folks."

"How's progress with the repairs?" Remy inquired.

"So far, so good. All the welding is done and the surveyor gave the thumbs-up. Once we sort out the painting, we'll be ready to launch- weather permitting-

which will probably be by the end of next week. The antifouling paint arrived yesterday. Seems like it gets pricier every time we need it," I grumbled.

"Don't forget, we've got a progress meeting on Friday morning. Can you have your checklist ready by then?" I asked Remy.

"Sure thing, John. I've gone over the survey report and the documents from the previous dry dock. We'll have everything lined up on Friday- assuming the interior decorator cooperates," Remy said with a smile.

"Another beer?" I offered.

"No, thanks, just the one for me. I've got dinner plans tonight with a lovely young lady who claims to be a fantastic chef. Just thinking ahead, John, you might need a new chef once we start chartering," Remy teased.

"Mmm, Remy, don't you see all those warning lights flashing? I've got enough on my plate right now; I don't need crew issues before we even set sail," I said, concern creasing my brow.

"Oh, before I forget, while going through the files, I noticed that Morning Mist underwent a refit in England at the yard where I used to work many years ago. If we need anything from them, I've got a good old friend there. It's always handy to know the history, I reckon. Anyway, I must get going, John. I'll catch up with you tomorrow," Remy said as he made his way down the stairs onto the quay.

I watched Remy descend, hoping the cradle would lower the yacht back into the water next week. I didn't fancy her staying out of the water for too long.

Finishing my beer, I followed the path Remy had taken, descending to the quay.

I paced slowly around the yacht, meticulously inspecting the sea inlet covers and mentally noting the anode connectors that needed replacing. I had a deep affection for the old yacht; it had been a significant part of my life for over twenty years.

Despite occasional disagreements with the owners; they had maintained their trust in me, awarding me the contract for the maintenance and management of the yacht for the next five years.

Morning Mist exuded a timeless charm. Designed before yachts adopted a bloated profile laden with excessive superstructure, she remained sleek and elegant, her lines conveying a sense of perpetual gracefulness. To me, she embodied the style of yacht I would have crafted for myself given the opportunity.

After completing my circuit around the hull, I climbed back up the stairs and jotted down some notes in my workbook.

It wasn't quite a diary, as I paid little heed to the dates. Instead, I filled one page and then seamlessly transitioned to the next, rendering entries and dates that were unrelated. Yet, amidst the organized chaos, I meticulously recorded all the important details- much to the surprise of suppliers and other business associates.

In the morning, I brewed a cup of coffee before the workers arrived. Today, I needed to ensure that they had all their materials sorted out because I would be occupied for most of the day with Sylvia and Remy. There was also the matter of the interior decorator to consider.

Sylvia would need to add her list of items to the schedule, which always seemed to grow closer to the launch date.

Remy arrived with Sylvia, the owner's agent and Primrose Harper, the young interior decorator, a little after nine.

"Ah, Sylvia, it's wonderful to see you. Welcome aboard," I greeted her warmly, giving her a gentle hug.

Extending a hand to Primrose, I continued, "Welcome aboard. I hope

Captain Remington has brought you up to speed about the refit. Perhaps you'd like to spend some time familiarizing yourself with the guest cabins and then join us in the dining saloon."

"Thank you, Mr. Hope. Yes, the Captain has briefed me about the yacht. I'm absolutely thrilled to be involved. I can't wait to explore the cabins. I have the drawings the Captain provided, so I'm confident I'll find my way around. I'll get back to you once I've given the cabins a thorough inspection," Primrose replied enthusiastically.

"Right, well, let's have a seat around the dining table; I'm eager to hear your updates, Sylvia. We need to secure some charters soon before the weather takes a turn; otherwise, I'll have the owners breathing down my neck again," I said, leading the way to the dining area.

The morning passed with Remy and me jotting down notes and deciding the program prior to the launch.

Sylvia was impressed by how seamlessly we worked together. We conversed fluently in the language of boats and equipment - although she found some of the terminology challenging to grasp.

Later, there was a soft tap on the door as Primrose asked hesitantly. "May I join you? I've finished inspecting all the cabins," she added.

"Of course," I said, rising from his seat to offer her a chair. "We'll need your input as soon as it's ready."

"Let's finalize the schedule here. Remy and Sylvia, is there anything else we need to add? Sylvia, could you gather the details from Primrose so we can organize the soft furnishings? Primrose, do you have anything to add from your end?" I asked.

"I'll need a day or two to check with the suppliers and then Sylvia and I can compile the orders. We've already agreed on the colors and style, so it shouldn't take too long after that," Primrose explained.

"We can handle that once we're back in the water, John" said Captain Remington "I suggest we leave it to Sylvia and Primrose as we have plenty to do" he added.

"Are we all set then?" Captain Remington inquired. "Feels like it's about time for lunch. Shall we head to the bistro for a bite to eat, ladies?"

"That sounds delightful. Primrose and I missed breakfast, so we're famished. Will you be joining us, John?" Sylvia asked.

"Sorry, I can't. I've got the guys here applying the paint primer. We're on a bit of a tight schedule with the drying times.

I need to ensure they proceed in the right order," I replied.

"Ah, what a shame. I'll swing by later this afternoon; I'd like to discuss charter prospects and pricing. Would around five work for you?" Sylvia suggested.

"Sounds perfect" I said, bidding them farewell.

Chapter 2
Charter Plans

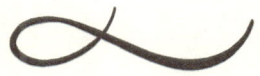

Just before five, I watched Sylvia return as she climbed the stairs from the quay.

Carrying a bright red briefcase, Sylvia epitomized elegance. I had known her for years, yet there was a line I hesitated to cross. I often pondered whether I should attempt to transition our relationship from friendship to something more.

"I've always admired your punctuality, Sylvia. Welcome back," I greeted her, offering my hand as she stepped aboard.

"It's the German in me, John. My parents were German and punctuality was instilled in me from an early age. It keeps things running smoothly," she explained before giving me a brief kiss on the cheek. "I could certainly use a cup of coffee, though. That was quite a long lunch."

"Sure thing, come on in and take a seat in the saloon. I'll get the coffee brewing. Black, no sugar, right?" I confirmed.

"Thanks, John. I'll get my questions ready. Primrose has a few concerns, and she's adamant about getting everything just right. so brace yourself. Importantly, I received a charter inquiry this afternoon for a five-day charter starting next weekend. Nothing like a bit of excitement to keep things interesting," Sylvia remarked with a smile.

I returned with a tray of coffee and biscuits. "Right, fire away, Sylvia," I said as I settled down next to her.

"Let's begin with the charter. Do you think we could pull it off? I know it's short notice. I mentioned it to Remy during lunch, and he seemed pretty confident, but wanted to wait until to discuss it with you," Sylvia suggested.

"Can we hold off on making a decision until Remy has had a look at things? I don't want to step on his toes, as he'd be taking responsibility for it. My gut feeling is that we should give it a shot. From the boat's perspective, we should be ready, but my main concern is the crew. We'll need to get that sorted out quickly, and that's definitely Remy's department," I concluded.

"That sounds reasonable, John. Let's review the various items we need to finalize," Sylvia agreed.

"Could you take charge of Primrose and the soft furnishings, Sylvia? I thought she showed great enthusiasm, and I'd hate to dampen that. She's young and, I suspect, a bit sensitive, and my usual bulldozer approach might not be the best fit for her," I requested.

"Of course, I can handle that, John. Do you want me to help sort out the crew as well?" Sylvia inquired.

"Yes please, if you could have a chat with Remy, that would be great. For this trip, I'll handle getting two deckhands and oversee the engine room. We'll also need a hostess and a chef. I know Remy has someone in mind" I confirmed.

"So, what should I tell the potential charter guests?" Sylvia asked.

"Let's meet tomorrow morning with Remy and make a final decision. I'll adjust the schedule and see if we can get the yacht back in the water earlier. If everything aligns, we can inform the guests, and if we secure their deposit, we'll proceed. Despite the short notice, I'm eager to resume chartering," I said.

"Sounds good. I'll speak with Remy tonight and arrange for us to meet for us all to meet tomorrow morning. Sylvia suggested.

"No need to worry. I'm meeting Remy for dinner at the yacht club this evening. You're welcome to join us. We can decide most of the matters over dinner," I suggested.

"Are you asking me out on a date, John?" Sylvia teased with a smile. "Always the romantic."

"I think Remy will be the one playing the romantic role with the potential chef. We can just chaperone him. I suspect he's invited her to dinner." I replied.

"It's been too long since we all had dinner together. I'd better head home and prepare for the evening. Anything else we need to sort out?" Sylvia inquired as we descended the stairs together, making our way across to her car.

"You really adore this old yacht, don't you, John? It's just like you in so many ways," Sylvia remarked as she climbed into her car. "See you at eight," she waved before driving off.

I returned to the boat and checked on the two painters as they wrapped up for the day.

"Hey, Justin, do you think you and the guys could work over the weekend to finish the painting and anti-fouling?" I asked. "I know it's short notice, but we might have a charter coming up and we are under pressure to finish sooner than planned."

"Sure thing. Each coat will only take a couple of hours, so we can do one tomorrow and the final coat on Sunday morning. If needed, I can bring in my two brothers to help paint as well". Justin, the elder of the two painters, assured me.

"I think that sounds like a plan, Justin. Bring them in tomorrow if you can and then we'll be sure to have the painting finished by Sunday," I decided.

After a refreshing shower, I dressed and made my way to the yacht club. The Caribbean night air was warm, and the shimmering lights danced across the water as I strolled along the promenade. Inside the club, Remy was seated at the bar, entertaining a couple of guests with tales that I was certain revolved around his island escapades.

"Evening, Captain," I greeted, extending my hand with a playful flourish.

"John, I was just talking about you. You haven't met Barbara, I believe," Remy said.

"Barbara, allow me to introduce you to the man I warned you about. Meet John Hope. There are plenty of stories about him, though only a handful that I'd feel comfortable sharing with you." Remy teased.

Barbara extended her hand to me. "I'm pleased to meet you, John. The captain was just recounting some of your adventures," she said with a warm smile.

I shook her hand and found myself captivated by her deep blue eyes, which were a mesmerizing blend of innocence and mischief. It was their sheer beauty that took my breath away.

"His stories are very one-sided, Barbara. You'll have to humor him," I remarked, reluctantly releasing her hand.

"A beer for you, John?" Remy offered with a knowing smile.

"Yes, please. I've got some interesting news for you. Sylvia will be joining us shortly. She's got a potential charter lined up for us, but we'll need to be ready by next Friday, if that's possible," I explained.

"Hmm, John, that's cutting it a bit close. It all hinges on when we can get the boat back in the water," Remy pondered.

"I've arranged for Justin and his painters to wrap things up over the weekend. If the weather holds, we can get her back in the water by Monday or Tuesday at the latest. I'll pick up the new anodes and fit them once the paint is dry," I said.

"What about the crew and the soft furnishings? We'll need to get those sorted out. A couple of sea trials wouldn't hurt before we start hosting guests. How many guests are we expecting, John?" Remy inquired.

"Let's wait to hear from Sylvia on that, Remy. As far as I know, there are just two guests, but we'll get the details from her," I replied.

As the bar filled with patrons, I spotted Sylvia entering through the doors. With a quip, I addressed Remy and Barbara, "Well, it's precisely eight o'clock. You can set your watches now – Sylvia has arrived."

Remy and I both stood up to welcome Sylvia.

"Sylvia," Remy greeted warmly, clasping both her hands, "You always bring a touch of elegance to the club. You look stunning. Please, allow me to introduce Barbara."

"It's a pleasure to meet you, Barbara," Sylvia acknowledged. "The Captain mentioned you're a chef. I've always admired those who are creative in the kitchen. Unfortunately, a poached egg is the extent of my culinary skills," she added with a smile.

"Sylvia, what would you like to drink?" I asked.

"I think I'll just have a glass of wine with dinner, John, if that's alright," Sylvia replied.

"Of course. Shall we proceed to dinner, Barbara?"

The dinner was delightfully casual, with tasty fresh seafood. Sylvia elaborated on the details of the potential charter and the necessary preparations. I allowed Sylvia and Remy to coordinate arrangements and plans for the charter. Meanwhile, I focused on making a mental to-do list of tasks. The next couple of days promised to be more than busy.

Justin and his brothers completed the final coat of antifouling in the afternoon. I inspected the hull with them, admiring how clean and fresh the boat looked with the new paint.

"Do you need a hand with the anodes, John? We can knock them out quickly if you want," Justin offered.

"That would be great. The spanners are with the new anodes. I also want to check the rudder. Those hydraulic guys can be a bit sloppy with the piping. I want to ensure they haven't mixed up the lines. Can you let me know what the rudder is doing if I give you a radio?" I asked.

I climbed the stairs and fetched a radio from the bridge, handing it to Justin. "Just tell me of the rudder's direction when I turn the wheel, Justin.

On the bridge, I radioed, "Justin, do you copy?" Justin responded that he did and the two of them checked that the rudder was working well.

"Affirmative, John. All looks spot on" Justin confirmed. "I'll bring the radio up to you," Justin replied.

Justin handed the radio back to me. I asked if he could join us as a deckhand if we secured the three-day charter. Justin was taking a navigation course so the sea miles would be good for him.

"It'll give you some sea miles towards your qualification. It's expected to be a short charter, three days tops, but I know you're eager," I offered. Justin thanked me and added that his brother had already finished a navigation course. I immediately offered him them both to join the charter – once it was confirmed.

"Thank you" said Justin "Things have been a bit slow lately, and my brother needs the extra cash to complete his skipper's course," added Justin with genuine gratitude.

"It'll be good to have you both onboard again. Tomorrow, we can start going over the systems," I said with a nod.

Once Justin and his brothers had departed, I found myself alone on the boat. I prepared a simple dinner for myself and savored a glass of wine, enjoying the tranquility.

Tomorrow, Remy and Sylvia would be joining me, along with Primrose. I wondered what Sylvia had arranged with Barbara. Part of me hoped Barbara would be joining the crew. Yet, I couldn't shake the realization that she was almost young enough to be my daughter.

40

Chapter 3
Crewing Up

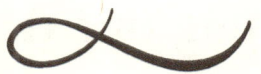

Monday morning proved as hectic as I had anticipated. The once silent vessel burst into life with Sylvia and Primrose meticulously inspecting linens, crockery and all other essentials for the upcoming charter.

Meanwhile, Remy as captain, stationed himself on the bridge to oversee equipment checks and the technicians who had come to adjust the angle of the newly-installed video camera on the aft rear deck - essential for docking maneuvers.

Justin and his brother had spent the morning cleaning out the storage areas and organizing the lines. They also took care of dropping the anchors and cleaning the chains.

By lunchtime, I was confident that 'Morning Mist' would be ready to return to the water the following day. The morning's high tide, just after ten, would make the process smoother.

I devoted most of the morning to the engine room, diligently going through my checklist. Despite the open portholes, the confined space was sweltering, so I stripped down to my blue shorts. As I finished, Justin appeared, poked his head in to announce that lunch was being served on the aft deck.

I washed my hands and ascended the stairs to the main deck. Joining the crew around the table, I noticed Primrose had brought her clipboard and was reviewing some items with Sylvia, who looked up as I approached.

"John, a shirt, please. We have standards to uphold. Shirts at mealtimes, please," Sylvia gently scolded, accompanied by a playful smile.

"Oh, I didn't realize we were going all formal now. I thought we could save that for when we're back in the water. It's sweltering down in the engine room," I defended myself.

"Can't take the docks out of him, Sylvia. Always a dockworker, just be thankful he has no tattoos," the Captain chimed in, enjoying my moment of discomfort.

As I pushed my chair back to rise, Barbara entered with a tray filled with lunch dishes. Placing the tray on the table, she reached for the shirt draped over her shoulder. "Here you are," she said with a warm smile. "You left it on the table in the crew quarters."

"Why, this looks delicious," Sylvia remarked, eagerly reaching for the bowls of fresh salad and steamed lobster—perfect for a summer day. "Thank you, Barbara, it's wonderful."

Sylvia hid a smile as she watched the satisfied looks between Remy and me. It was evident that Barbara had passed the test to be chef. Along with Primrose for guest services, the crew was now complete.

Conversation around the lunch table revolved around the scheduled launch for the following morning. Sylvia confirmed that the charter deposit had been sent and anticipated confirmation by the end of the business day.

"The charter group was originally four people, but one couple has had to cancel, so it's just the one couple now," Sylvia said. "Primrose has nearly finished with the forward cabin—it's the nicest one and looks stunning. We can add some fresh flowers as a final touch just before we depart. John, come and have a look after lunch. I think you'll approve."

Primrose and Sylvia were in the final stages of completing the soft furnishings for the lounge area and planned to have the final deliveries on board by Thursday.

"Remy, can we gather together this afternoon with Jason and Gideon, his brother? I want everyone to be clear on what's expected. How about around four? It shouldn't take more than half an hour. Oh, by the way, Sylvia, have the guests made any requests for places they'd like to visit around the Bahamas?" I inquired.

"I'll check with them as soon as I receive the deposit," Sylvia replied.

"See if you can sell them on Norman's Cay and Shroud Cay," Remy suggested. "If they're interested in snorkeling, those are two excellent spots not too far."

"Will do, Remy," Sylvia said.

I then spent time with Sylvia and Primrose finalizing arrangements for the housekeeping including new china, cutlery and glasses. They agreed that a tour a little later would enable me to check all the work they had completed.

In truth, my mind was busy with other things.

"Now, about tomorrow", I said getting their attention. "We'll be going back in the water starting around nine". I then carefully explained what this would mean in reality as no one would be able to get on or off the boat for two hours and that there would be no power onboard during the launch. I suggested that they all planned what they would do for the morning and that it would be the ideal time to go into town for supplies.

"Sorry to interrupt," said Primrose shyly, "I think Sylvia and I have forgotten about the crew uniforms. We need to get the sizes needed for everyone," Primrose added.

"Best to get a couple of extra shirts for John here too" Sylvia quipped, jesting with me.

Chapter 4
Launching

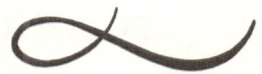

I MADE myself a cup of coffee early that Tuesday morning. I watched the deckhands greasing the blocks ready for launching the yacht. I was grateful to have the two brothers as crew.

Both of them made up for what they lacked in experience with boundless enthusiasm and were always keen to lend a hand.

I had just placed my empty cup in the galley when Captain Remington arrived on the quay. I hurried down the stairs to join him.

"Looks like we're all set, Remy. The deposit is in the account." We walked around the hull for a final inspection with the brothers.

"Are all the sea intakes clean, Justin?" Captain Remington asked. "Have you turned the props?"

"It's all done, Captain. We turned the props yesterday; everything is ready from here. All the valves are closed for the sea intakes," confirmed Justin.

"Good. Remember to close all the portholes before we launch" said Captain Remington " I know it's a pain, but if we don't and something goes wrong, the insurers will ask many questions."

"We'll do that, Captain. The lines are ready on deck, and we have set up the fenders on both sides," Justin explained with pride.

It looks like we're all set then, I thought to myself. It will be marvelous getting back on the water and sailing together – it has been far too long. I knew that Sylvia would be bringing Primrose and Barbara along. They all want to be on board for the launch, so as soon as they get here, we will go. I smiled to myself with this prospect.

Sylvia arrived a little after nine along with Barbara and Primrose wearing their new crew uniforms. Captain Remington and I looked on admiringly before we did our final checks in the engine room.

"We've got about two hundred gallons of fuel in the day tank". I told Remy. "I've checked the hydraulic levels, and they're fine. The compressors are up to pressure, so we're ready to go, Remy," I said confidently, giving him a friendly pat on his shoulder.

"We've got a good crew here, I remarked. "I'm looking forward to this trip."

I handed out the handheld radios to Justin and his brother and kept one for myself. "Check your radios, guys, make sure you can talk to the captain. Justin, you're on the port side; Gideon, you're on starboard. Make sure you're close to the fenders. The wind will push us towards the platform arms on the starboard side."

There was one remaining radio and I took it to the aft deck where Barbara and Primrose stood. I gave them a quick lesson how to use a marine radio and demonstrated how quickly I could speak to Justin using it.

I handed the radio to Barbara. "If you see anything that doesn't look right, quickly tell us on the radio.

I went up to the bridge and joined Remy. The winch operator stood ready at the winch, and I held up my radio to let him know we were ready.

I held up my radio to let the marine engineers on the quayside know we were ready. The shore power to the yacht was disconnected.

The boat cradle gave a slight jolt as the slack in the thick wire ropes was taken up and the safety clamps were released. All was looking good.

I asked if we could stop about a foot above the water so I could start the engines and agreed that the rubber duck inflatable dinghy should be close by on standby.

The yacht was slowly but surely moved to a position above the water. "Remy, I'm off to the engine room" I said finding it hard to contain my excitement. I reached for my radio. "Keep an eye on the depth and make sure we stop when we're a foot off floating" I reminded everyone over the radio.

I opened the sea inlet valves for the main engines in the engine room.

"Right, John, we should have enough water now; you want to start up?" inquired Remy over the radio.

I switched on the generator and started both engines. The main engines growled, and it felt like the boat had suddenly come back to life. I carefully checked the oil pressure, and once I was sure all was well, I climbed up the stairs back to the bridge.

"We're all set, Remy; let the shore crew know we can go, please," I said.

Remy relayed the message over the radio and thanked them for their hard work.

"On your way, Captain" came the prompt reply. "You have seven feet of water now. Safe travels."

The bow of the yacht slowly rose as the boat gained buoyancy, settling into its natural position in the water. The two deckhands secured the lines as the yacht began to drift away from the platform.

"Are we all clear?" Captain Remington's voice crackled over the radio.

"Just a sec, Remy, I'm just double-checking," I replied.

Suddenly, Primrose's voice came over the radio. "Hey, not sure if this is a big deal, but there's something black floating at the back of the boat. It looks like a huge net or something similar."

I quickly grabbed my radio. "Remy, don't go astern. We've picked up something at the back of the boat. I'm going to check. Gideon and Justin, don't let your lines go. Stand by," I urgently relayed.

Racing to the aft deck where Primrose and Barbara were leaning over the bulwark, I leaned over beside them to see a pallet with netting attached to it floating next to the rudder. I reached for my radio again.

I called out over the radio to the engineers on land.

"Yes, John, what's the problem?" responded Eddie, the boss.

"We've picked up some debris on the stern. It looks like maybe a pallet with netting. Can you send someone to retrieve it?" I requested.

"Understood, John. We'll get someone out there right away," Eddie confirmed.

As I waited for assistance to arrive, I kept a watchful eye on the situation, ensuring the safety of the crew and the yacht.

The rubber duck inflatable dinghy arrived and quickly attached a line to the problem netting. With a bit of effort, the pallet and netting came free - much to my relief. I had been concerned that the netting might catch on the rudder or props, but thankfully, everything seemed clear.

"Alright, Remy, let's reverse; I think we've had enough excitement for one day," I said, relieved. "Gideon, Justin, reel in the lines, please."

As the propellers churned the water astern, the boat slowly moved backward and soon found itself in the channel.

"Great job, everyone," I radioed. "Could the fenders be moved over to the port side? We'll be tying up on the port side."

A few minutes after eleven, "Morning Mist" was safely moored alongside the quay. With her protective fenders out and lines neatly stowed, she looked almost majestic with her bright new paintwork.

I wiped the sweat off my forehead as I shut the engines down. The generator would have to keep humming until we had connected the shore power. Despite the drama, I couldn't hide my happiness.

As I made my way to the galley for a drink, Sylvia intercepted me in the passageway. "You look like the cat that got the cream, John. I can see that you are in your element; it's quite attractive. Oh, drinks are served on the aft deck, and for once, you don't need a shirt," she added with a smile. "By the way, I'm very impressed. Well done."

Captain Remington raised his glass to me. "Well done, John. It's fantastic to be back on the water, and the crew – you guys were all excellent. Primrose, you were truly great. Thank you for being so observant. You have the sweetest voice I've ever heard on a marine radio."

Sylvia and Primrose spent the afternoon organizing the remaining items, while Justin and his brother Gideon, checked the dinghy and crane on the upper deck.

Remy and I found ourselves alone on the aft deck, tasked with sorting out the accommodations. Justin and his brother were set to move aboard, sharing one of the crew cabins. Barbara and Primrose would each have their own crew cabin, while Sylvia would occupy one of the guest cabins. I would take up residence in the aft guest cabin and Remy would settle himself into the captain's cabin.

"Our guests can take the forward Stateroom," I suggested. "It's the largest cabin on the boat and Primrose has truly outdone herself with the upgrades. She's got some serious talent and that angelic face of hers doesn't hurt either. I'm grateful Sylvia invited her to join us. She really saved the day earlier."

"Are you game for a short sea trial tomorrow morning, John?" Remy inquired. "I'd like Justin and Gideon to take the helm for a bit, just so they're familiar with doing so, in case of any emergencies."

"Let's aim for early, maybe around seven," I suggested. "We only need about an hour or so and then we can return. I know Sylvia will want to grab some last-minute supplies, leaving us a clear day before the guests arrive."

"I'm excited about this," Remy admitted. "We're going to have a blast chartering this old yacht. She's a real beauty."

Chapter 5
Charter Guests

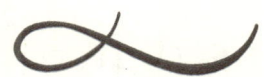

THE DAY before our guests arrived onboard flew by in a whirlwind of activity. Having completed all my preparation work, I felt restless as I double-checked every detail, fretting in case I might have overlooked something.

The brothers and I practised lowering the dinghy into the water and ensuring the crane was in good working order. Meanwhile, Primrose added her final touches to the Forward Stateroom. I was amazed by the level of detail she put into it. She even consulted Sylvia to determine the guests' flower preferences, resulting in a vase of vibrant orange Birds of Paradise flowers tastefully arranged in the saloon and another smaller one in the Stateroom.

Barbara took charge of the guests' food preferences, spending more time than I deemed necessary to create the menu for the three-day excursion, working closely with Sylvia throughout.

Captain Remington spent the afternoon with me going over the itinerary, Remy explained. "So, these guys want to do quite a bit of snorkeling. I'd suggest we spend a day at Norman's Cay. It's a short sail down to the

Exumas, and they can spend their time snorkeling or, if they're up for it, diving to explore the WWII plane wreckage just offshore."

He continued, "Remember that beautiful sheltered beach just south of the wreck? The one we visited with the group from Germany? They didn't want to leave. We can anchor there for the night, and if they fancy going ashore for dinner, there's that restaurant with the amazing grill."

"Should we also include Shroud Cay, Remy?" I pondered. "I've always been fond of the 'washing machine' current, but I'm not sure if they'd enjoy it. Maybe we should offer a couple of alternatives after their day snorkeling at Norman's."

"You're right. I'm not sure if it's their first trip here, so let's see what they want to do," Remy agreed.

I entertained the idea of taking a short nap before dinner, but I had barely settled onto my bunk when there came a tap on the door. "Mind if I interrupt you for a few minutes, John? I need to sort out the contracts for the crew," Sylvia said.

"Of course, come on in Sylvia, let's take a look at what you've got," I replied.

Sylvia handed me the contracts for the crew.

"You'll need to sign all the contracts for the crew, but remember, I don't have one. I'm a guest, so you'll have to be extra kind to me, John," Sylvia joked.

"Always, Sylvia. You've done an outstanding job. I'm not sure I would've agreed to the charter without you around," I assured her.

"There is one thing I should mention, John. When you have a chance, please take a look at Barbara's resume and let me know what you think. Maybe I'm overreacting, but hey, better safe than sorry. Have a look and let me know, John," Sylvia added.

"I'll do that, Sylvia. What do you know about the guests?" I inquired.

"Not much info on them, John; it's a referral from another charter company that couldn't take the booking. They seem to be in their late thirties, pretty active. They're into beach days and snorkeling. No weird food requests, just your standard gin and tonic preferences. I'll have to get Remy to charm some details out of them," Sylvia said as she gathered the contracts. "Sorry for the interruption; dinner's at seven. You know the dress code, right?" She grinned.

That evening we all ate together. It was Captain Remy who suggested the crew dining together when the guests weren't around would give Primrose and Barbara a chance to get the hang of boat lingo.

After dinner, Captain Remy went over the charter details. "Tomorrow, the guests are arriving around nine, so Barbara, let's keep it simple with coffee, fruit juices, and maybe a few snacks. Oh, and some little cakes too."

He continued, "We'll give them time to settle in, then set sail at ten to reach Norman's Cay by lunchtime. I imagine they will want to get in the water soon after lunch. Weather's forecasted to be in the low nineties, so it's gonna be hot. Gideon and Justin, make sure the dinghy's good to go once we arrive. Let's hit the sack early and be ready for tomorrow. I'm dead set on having fun with this charter, and I want all of you to have a great time. Let's do everything we can to give the guests the best vacation."

After the table was cleared, Sylvia and I found ourselves alone on the aft deck.

"I went through Barbara's resume, Sylvia. Did you check her references?" I inquired.

"No, I tried, but I couldn't reach her previous employer with the number she provided," Sylvia replied.

"It might be nothing, but those employment gaps and frequent job changes are concerning. We don't have any other options now, so let's keep a close watch. I'm calling it a night. Tomorrow's going to be, how do you say it... ereignisreich?" I remarked.

"Eventful, John. Stick to English. Your German pronunciation is terrible," Sylvia teased.

Paula and Steve MacMaster arrived just before nine-thirty in the morning. Captain Remington greeted them on the quay, looking immaculate in his captain's uniform, flanked by Gideon and Justin, ready to assist with their bags and cases. I observed him from one of the engine room portholes, admiring Remy's refined style.

Onboard, Sylvia introduced Primrose and Barbara to the MacMasters and escorted them to their stateroom.

"Oh, this is absolutely wonderful!" exclaimed Paula MacMaster. "Isn't it just lovely, Stevie?" she whispered.

"Fantastic!" exclaimed Steve, pushing his sunglasses up onto his closely cropped hair.

"Please, take your time to get settled. We have some refreshments on the aft deck. Primrose will show you. We're scheduled to depart at ten. If there's anything you need, just let us know," Sylvia said in her most hospitable tone.

I started the generator and ascended the stairs to the bridge. "We're all set to go, Remy. Shore power can be disconnected and Justin and Gideon are ready," I reported.

"Right on, John, just give me two minutes. I need to radio in and get the chart plotter set up. You can fire up the engines if you like," Remy said.

With the main engines running, I returned to the bridge to ensure all instruments were functioning properly. "All looks good, Remy. I'll go help

Gideon and Justin. I'll keep an ear out on the radio," I confirmed.

I made my way along the port side. Remy came over the radio, "Alright, John, can you please have the guys bring in the lines? Prepare to go astern a bit. I need some space to clear the quay."

Slowly, the boat shifted astern, then turned and smoothly moved ahead, heading out into the channel.

"Aah this is John Hope, our engineer on the yacht. John, meet Steve and Paula MacMaster," Sylvia introduced the couple as I reached out to shake their hands. "Welcome onboard, both of you. I hope you have a wonderful time. We should arrive at Norman's Cay around lunchtime. The weather's great, so it should be a comfortable trip. Have you been shown around the yacht yet?"

"We've seen our lovely room, John; it's absolutely gorgeous. Primrose gave us a tour," Paula replied.

"Great, well, enjoy yourselves. I'll see you when we reach Norman's Cay. We'll drop anchor there and the crew will launch the dinghy so you can head to the beach or go snorkeling. There are also two kayaks available. Just let the crew know. Justin and Gideon are both experienced open-water divers, and they'd be happy to show you around," I informed them.

I joined Captain Remington on the bridge as the boat cruised gracefully through the water at eight knots. "The boat loves this speed, John. Engines are at just about nine hundred rpm. She feels perfectly balanced," Remy remarked. "It's great being back on board with you."

"The guests seem content enough. We should reach Norman's around half past one for lunch, and then they can go snorkeling or whatever they fancy," I replied.

After lunch, Paula and Steve waited on the aft deck for Gideon to bring the two kayaks around. Covered in sunscreen and sporting bright fins and new goggles, they were eager to hit the water. Paula complained that the strap on her goggles was too tight, so Steve adjusted it for her.

When Captain Remington saw the kayaks in the water, he called Justin. "You better get the dinghy in the water and take Gideon with you. Those folks don't look too steady on the kayaks."

Primrose hurried to the aft deck as Justin lowered the dinghy into the water. Sylvia had agreed that Primrose could join the brothers in the dinghy, and it seemed they were happy to have her along.

The afternoon passed calmly onboard. Sylvia, Remy, and I sat on the aft deck, watching Paula and Steve enjoy the clear water. Later, Barbara brought us drinks as we observed the dinghy slowly towing the kayaks toward the beach.

"Looks like the guests have had their fill of water," Remy remarked. "Sylvia, could you ask Barbara to prepare a couple of drinks for them? I'll call Justin to come pick them up. They'll also need some towels."

The dinghy returned to the yacht as the sun began to set. The brothers stowed the kayaks and hoisted the dinghy back onto the upper deck. The guests looked a little sunburned and tired, and they were eager to turn in after an early dinner.

Chapter 6
The Missing Diamond

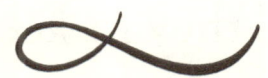

IN THE early morning on the bridge, I scrolled through the weather report. A light north-easterly wind was forecast, and the temperature would be a more moderate eighty-five degrees. It looked to be another perfect day for sailing around the Bahamas.

"We never got a chance to chat with Steve and Paula about their plans for today. I'm thinking we head up to Shroud Cay. It's a relaxed cruise, and I've tentatively booked a mooring if needed. What do you think Remy?" I asked.

"We could make a stop at Hawksbill Cay on the way if they're keen and maybe spot some turtles" suggested Remy before continuing "I doubt they're adventurous enough to swim with the sharks at Compass Cay.

Why don't you talk to them over breakfast, I suggested,' You are the gracious host, remember?" I chuckled.

"Morning," Sylvia said as she entered the bridge, looking rather flustered. "We have a problem downstairs. It seems Paula has misplaced her diamond pendant. Steve apparently gave it to her as a tenth wedding anniversary gift last month."

Sylvia continued anxiously, "She doesn't know its value because Steve is too afraid to tell her how valuable it is. Paula claims she left it in their Stateroom yesterday, but this morning, it is nowhere to be found." Sylvia spoke quickly, stress evident in her voice.

"I need to speak with the couple urgently. We need to resolve this; something like this could be very detrimental to the boat's reputation," she concluded.

"Have you asked Primrose and Barbara if they've been in the Stateroom?" I asked.

"No, I came straight up here after talking to Paula. She's terribly upset and angry. She says unless they find the diamond, they want to head straight back to Nassau," Sylvia reported.

"Alright, I'll see what I can do," I replied. "Can you have a chat with Primrose and Barbara? Maybe separately would be better. See if they can shed any light on it."

"Sure, I will. The MacMasters are on the rear aft deck having coffee," Sylvia replied.

" Actually, on second thoughts, it's best I handle it" I said. "I'll have a word with Barbara, if you don't mind. I've been replaying yesterday afternoon in my mind. Justin and Gideon were on the dinghy with Primrose while Barbara was inside the boat. She prepared the drinks and snacks while they were all on the beach."

I ran my fingers through my hair. "Just what we didn't need right now," I said wearily, making my way down from the bridge.

"John," Sylvia quickly called me, "there's something else that is worrying me. I overheard Primrose thanking Barbara last night for placing fresh towels in the

MacMasters' cabin. Primrose had forgotten when she hurried to join the brothers on the dinghy, so Barbara took them into the MacMasters' cabin yesterday afternoon," Sylvia added with concern.

"Hmm, let's not jump to conclusions just yet. Circumstances have a way of surprising us. Let's get Barbara up here and see what she can tell us," I suggested.

Barbara listened as I informed her of the missing diamond pendant. She struggled to hold back the tears that welled up in her eyes when she realized she was being viewed with suspicion.

"I know we haven't had much time to get to know each other, John, and I'm truly grateful for this job, but I can't even imagine what the diamond pendant looks like. I haven't seen it, and I'm shocked that this has happened. All I can say is, if you want to search my cabin, Sylvia is welcome to go through all my bags," Barbara said sadly.

"Barbara, I don't want to search your cabin. I just need you to understand that this charter is crucial for the yacht and all the crew. We can't afford an incident like this tarnishing the excellent service we provide. Our jobs are on the line now, so please, if there's anything you need to tell us, now's the time," I said.

"John, I needed this job more than anything. I would never do anything to jeopardize it, especially since you, Sylvia, and everyone else on the boat have been so kind to me. I'm sorry," she stammered before breaking down in tears.

Sylvia gently hugged Barbara. "Don't worry, we'll figure this out, one way or another. Barbara, let's go downstairs and get something to drink."

Left alone on the silent bridge, I recalled refitting it last year, replacing all the old and obsolete equipment with new navigation plotting computers and modern radios. I couldn't help but think it was a pity we hadn't installed security cameras in the staterooms and cabins too. It would have made solving the mystery much simpler. Ummm, that gave me an idea.

On the new video screen that I had installed to aid with reverse astern maneuvers, I could observe part of the aft deck where Remy engaged in a serious conversation with Steve and Paula. Out of curiosity, I checked the controls. The system had automatically recorded the past twenty-four hours, so I scrolled through the timeline to yesterday afternoon when Paula and Steve were preparing to kayak.

I replayed the footage from the moment Steve assisted Paula getting into the kayak. Paula was clad in a bright red bikini and hat adorned with a matching red ribbon and appeared somewhat unsteady in the kayak. As she reached up to take the paddle from Steve, I stared in disbelief. The diamond pendant was unmistakably visible around her neck. My view was quickly obscured as Steve joined her in the kayak. I re-wound the video to confirm my observation. There it was, glinting in the sunlight. I paused the video, zoomed in and used the 'take a picture' function to capture a photograph of the scene.

"Now," I thought, "if I can just find the moment when they return back to the boat." I fast-forwarded until Gideon appeared on the screen, securing the dinghy for Barbara and Steve to embark.

Steve boarded the yacht first, offering Barbara a hand as she followed. Although her face and neck were obscured by her hat, when she turned to reach for the towel basket, I saw clearly. There was no pendant. I captured another photograph. It looked like I had the evidence we needed.

I switched off the video screen and climbed down the stairs to the lower deck to find Sylvia in the galley. "Is Barbara okay Sylvia?" I asked.

"Unless she's an outstanding actress, I really don't think she knows anything about the diamond. She's terribly upset," Sylvia replied.

"Would you mind going to her and telling her that everything is sorted out? She doesn't have to worry at all," I requested.

"What's happened? Have you found the diamond, John?" Sylvia asked in surprise.

"It's all good, Sylvia, but first please tell Barbara not to worry. I'm going to talk with Steve and Paula." I assured her.

"Morning, Steve, Paula. I'm so sorry to hear about your pendant," I said kindly as I addressed the couple.

"We're more than sorry," Steve responded solemnly. "It was my gift to Paula for our tenth wedding anniversary. I can't express how special it was. We'd like to head back to Nassau as soon as possible. We're considering having the police meet us on the quay to search the crew cabins. We'll need to get a crime number for the insurance company."

It was clear from his voice that he was both angry and frustrated.

"However, Captain Remington has advised us that the yacht has its own insurance, so I hope that will cover you for the cost of the diamond, although the sentimental value will never be recovered," Steve concluded.

"That would be very disappointing for all of us, Steve. We had a great itinerary planned, but I understand your position. I'll get the boat ready to head for home straight away. We're not more than two hours away." My voice was confident and re-assuring.

"Again, I'm very sorry to ask you one last time, but are you absolutely sure that the diamond was left in your cabin while you went kayaking yesterday?" I asked, looking Steve straight in the eye.

"Please, this is totally unacceptable" exclaimed Paula. I treasured that diamond more than anything. I would very well know where I kept it. It's just a pity there was no safe storage in the cabin. I would have locked it away," Paula said rather bitterly.

"Well, I'll get the engines fired up, and we can head back. It's an unfortunate situation," I replied calmly.

Before I began preparing to start the engines, Remy joined me in the engine room.

"You're a little casual about events John. They're going to hold us responsible for their loss," Remy remarked.

"Not so, Remy. Let me get the engines up and running, and then I'll show you some interesting things on the bridge," I said with a conspiratorial wink.

When we were both on the bridge, I switched on the video screen. Paula and Steve were still engrossed in conversation on the aft deck.

"Have a look at this, Remy, its from yesterday," I said as I switched to the photographs I had taken from the video. "Here's the first one, Paula in the kayak. You can see the diamond pendant clearly?"

"Wow, yes, that means she had the pendant on when they went kayaking. It wasn't in the cabin as she thought." Remy observed.

"Right," I said, "but have a look at this photo from when they got back." I flipped to the next screenshot. "No pendant."

"So she either lost it while kayaking or when they were on the beach, but the pendant couldn't have been on the yacht as she thought.

"Why didn't you mention this to Steve or Paula when we were all on the aft deck?" Remy asked.

"Because I think they set this up. I'm not sure about the value of the diamond. I suspect that Steve gave Paula an inflated value to cover up some debts he needed to pay. I'm keen to see if they really will call the cops to meet us on the quay. He will have to show some proof of valuation for the diamond, which may be uncomfortable for him. I bet you a case of beers that Steve will be offering to make a deal before we get to the quay," I speculated.

"Sailing with you is never boring, John." said Remy shaking his head in disbelief.

"Let's get these engines running." I commanded." I want this couple off the boat as soon as possible. Homeward bound at maximum speed, please, you old sea dog."

Remy responded with a huge grin.

Epilogue
All's Well

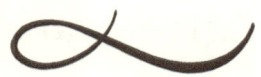

I PRINTED the two photographs I had taken as evidence and placed them in a padded envelope.

My prediction proved accurate. Steve approached the bridge about half an hour before we reached Nassau.

He proposed a deal where the yacht's insurance could resolve the issue by paying them half the implied value of the diamond pendant. Ten thousand dollars would make the problem of the missing diamond pendant go away with no repercussions for the yacht's crew and no police on the quay.

Captain Remington stared him down.

Once the yacht had tied up, Steve approached Captain Remington again, suggesting that in the absence of any payment, the police should be called after all.

Captain Remington told Steve that would not be wise and called me over.

"Mr. Hope has an envelope for you," he said to Steve. "The crew is ready to take your bags onto the quayside. Perhaps that would be the appropriate place for you to open the envelope and view its contents. I believe we've settled the matter."

Thinking the envelope contained the payment, Steve eagerly took the envelope and along with Paula, followed their bags onto the quay.

The crew watched with satisfaction as Steve opened the envelope and glanced in horror at the photographs. Paula snatched them from his hand and hurled them at the yacht before they hastily made their way to their waiting taxi.

I felt a tender arm around my shoulders. "I don't know how to thank you enough," whispered Barbara.

The End

Other Books from Seniorality

To find your next book John Hope book visit:

www.amazon.com/author/seniorality

Where you will find:

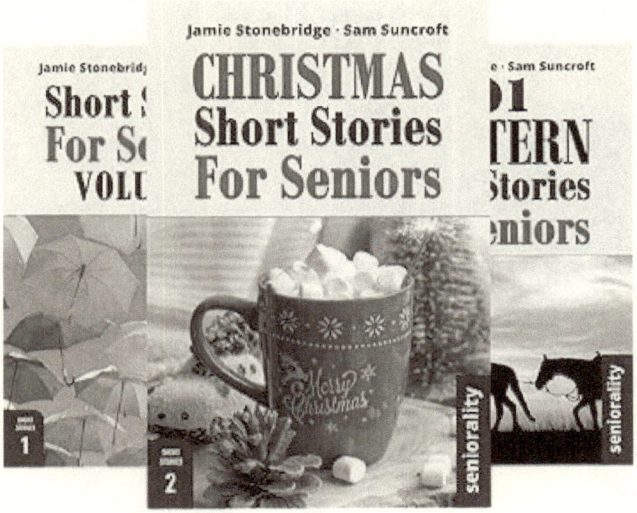

Short Stories

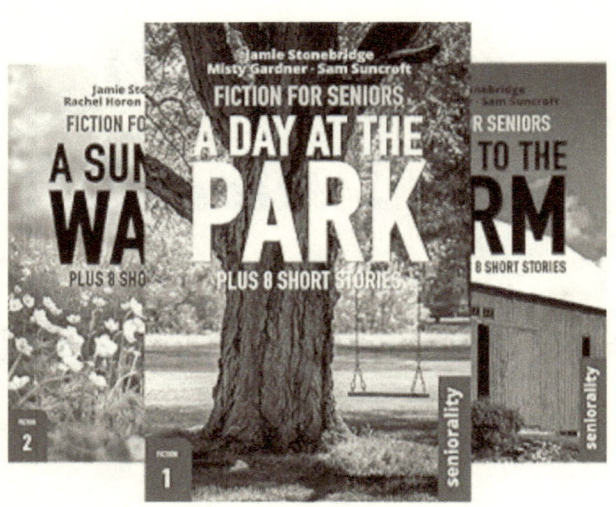

Fiction for Seniors

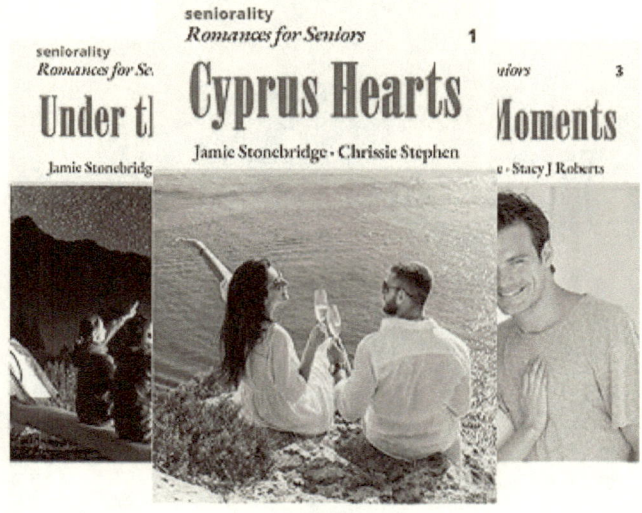

Romances for Seniors

Find these books and many more
by searching on Amazon for

'seniorality'

or visit:

www.amazon.com/author/seniorality

Thank You

If you enjoyed this book or found it useful, we'd be very grateful if you'd write a short review on Amazon.

Your support really does make a difference and helps other people discover this book.

We personally read all reviews to hear how the books are being used, to collect feedback, and get ideas for future stories.

Thank you and have a wonderful day!

www.ingramcontent.com/pod-product-compliance
Lightning Source LLC
Chambersburg PA
CBHW020442220526
45464CB00002B/821